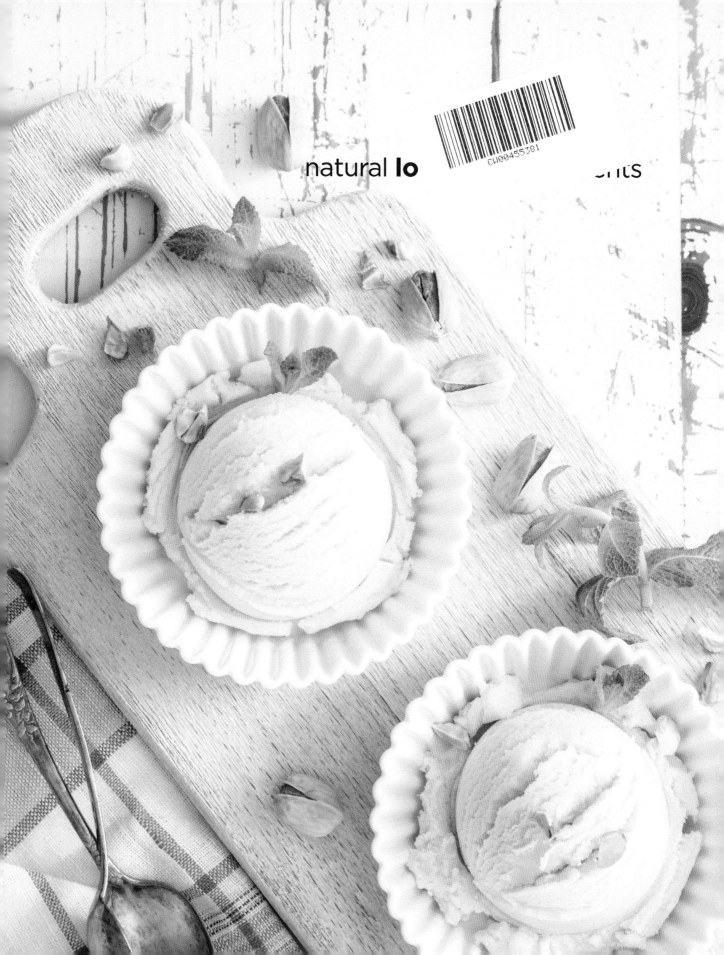

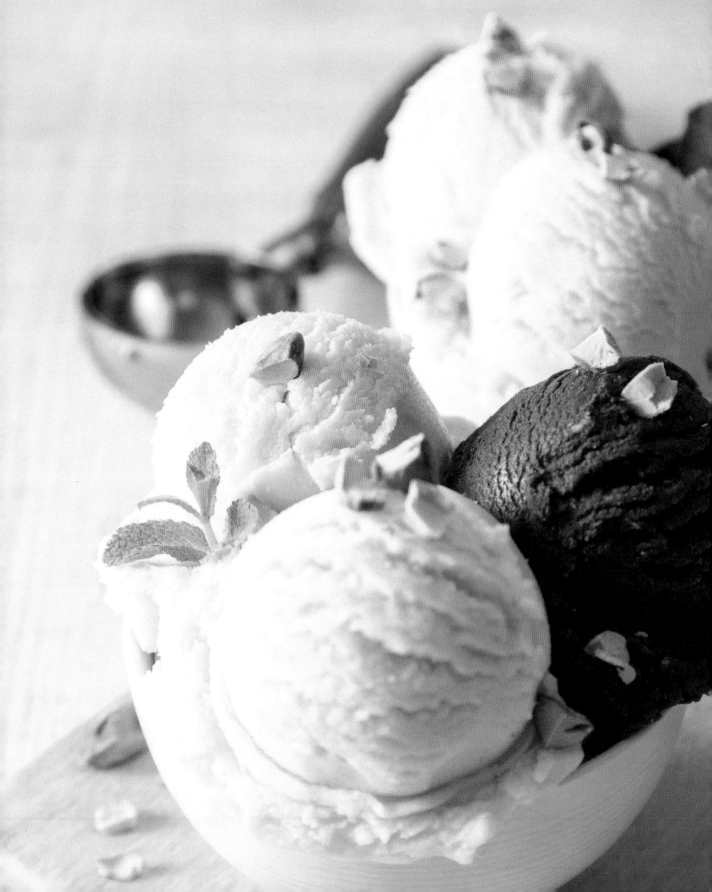

Life is like an ice cream, **enjoy** it before it melts

It is finally summer and, if like me, you are missing some good old-fashioned ice cream, then this book is the answer for you (even if you are not on a low-carb diet). This book is a compilation of my 20 most loved, most requested ice cream recipes that anyone can easily recreate.
All the recipes listed in this book are:

INTRODUCTION

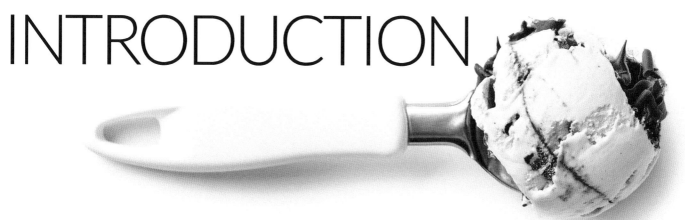

- **Easy** - Nobody has time for recipes that take hours and hours and hours

- **Low-Carb** - Each one has a net carb content of less than 10 g

- **High Fat** - Contain natural fat-rich ingredients

- **Customizable** - Don't like an ingredient? Substitute it for another!

- **Delicious-** This one is a given

- Can be made with or without an ice cream maker (there is a guide inside)

I hope you enjoy the recipes and they help you on your journey to a healthier and fitter you.

Elizabeth

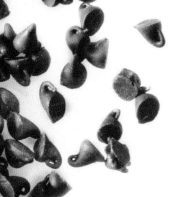

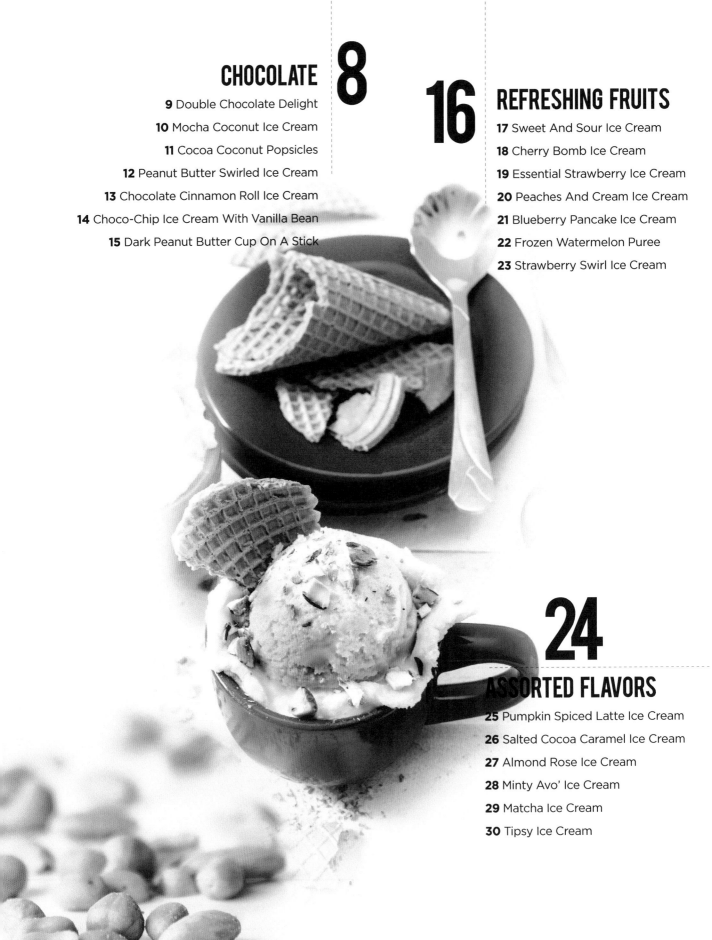

CHOCOLATE 8

9 Double Chocolate Delight
10 Mocha Coconut Ice Cream
11 Cocoa Coconut Popsicles
12 Peanut Butter Swirled Ice Cream
13 Chocolate Cinnamon Roll Ice Cream
14 Choco-Chip Ice Cream With Vanilla Bean
15 Dark Peanut Butter Cup On A Stick

16 REFRESHING FRUITS

17 Sweet And Sour Ice Cream
18 Cherry Bomb Ice Cream
19 Essential Strawberry Ice Cream
20 Peaches And Cream Ice Cream
21 Blueberry Pancake Ice Cream
22 Frozen Watermelon Puree
23 Strawberry Swirl Ice Cream

24 ASSORTED FLAVORS

25 Pumpkin Spiced Latte Ice Cream
26 Salted Cocoa Caramel Ice Cream
27 Almond Rose Ice Cream
28 Minty Avo' Ice Cream
29 Matcha Ice Cream
30 Tipsy Ice Cream

SWEET TALK

Before we begin and start talking about the different recipes, I'd like to take a moment to talk about the substitute sweeteners that we will be using.

Even people who are not on the ketogenic diet have come around to knowing the dangers of white sugar. Some people even refer to it as "white poison." Combine this with the rise in diabetes and weight gain problems, sugar substitutes have spiraled up in popularity in the past few decades.

Now there are many different sugar substitutes, and they come under various brand names, but in this book, I have used only two, stevia and erythritol, because they are the safest and have the most natural flavor.

Now you might notice that some recipes call for stevia while others call for erythritol, and there are some that need both. There is a science behind that.

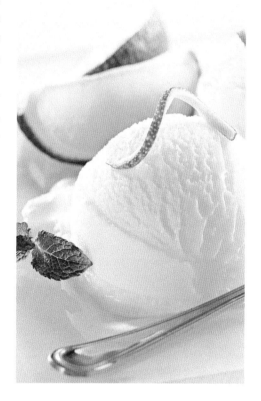

Stevia, or stevia extract as it should be called, is the extract of the stevia plant which occurs naturally. It is a zero calorie sweetener so is perfect for our needs. In the market, it either comes in liquid or powder form. Both are fine. Powder form is more suited for use in cakes and baking while liquid is more suited for liquid-y recipes such as smoothies. In the ice cream recipes listed in the book, liquid stevia is recommended.

Erythritol, on the other hand, is a naturally-occurring substance that is found in some fruits and cheeses. Like stevia, it is also calorie free. However, one distinction between the two is that erythritol gives a glazed appearance to the dishes hence making it perfect for icings, coatings and yes, ice cream! Using erythritol will give your ice cream a gelato-like look. Also, erythritol is a grain to grain sugar substitute which means that one tablespoon of white sugar and one tablespoon of erythritol will give the same amount of sweetness so using it is very easy.

Both are safe, heat-stable and taste neutral. It is a good idea to have them both in your pantry. Preferably have some liquid stevia and granulated erythritol on hand, but if you have to choose, I'd suggest that you go with erythritol because it is more versatile and is easier to use despite being a little more pricey.

I hope that this cleared up the common confusion about non-calorie sweeteners. So let's get started.

NO ICE-CREAM MAKER, NO PROBLEM!

Like everything in the kitchen, having the right tools for the job makes it life that much easier, but where there is a will (and an Internet) there is a way.

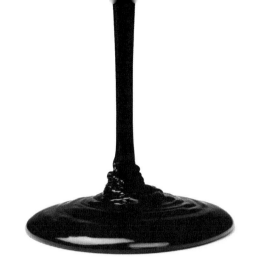

I know how my mum taught me to make ice cream, however, I was not convinced that it was the easiest method, so I tried a few different ideas from the internet to see if there was a better method... perhaps unsurprisingly, there were a lot. I tried a variety of techniques, but have to give credit to 'tasteofhome.com', which was the easiest and also the most compatible with my recipes.

While using an electric or hand-cranked ice cream maker will get you to your sweet reward a little easier, it's not a necessity.

Here's how to make do without one:

- Combine the ingredients for your ice cream mixture following the recipe. Chill the mixture over an ice bath. Meanwhile, freeze an empty freezer-safe shallow bowl or pan. Stainless steel works well for this.

- Place the cold mixture into the cold pan.

- Chill for about 20 minutes and check your ice cream. As the edges start to freeze, stir the mixture rapidly with a whisk or spatula to break up the partially frozen ice cream.

- This will help make it smooth and creamy. You cannot over-beat. Return to the freezer.

- Stir ice cream vigorously every 30 minutes until it is firmly frozen. This may be repeated

- 4 to 5 times until mixture is smooth and creamy. If ice cream becomes too hard, place it into the refrigerator until it becomes soft enough to beat and continue the process.

- Ripen the ice cream by storing it in a covered freezer container until ready to serve.

http://www.tasteofhome.com/recipes/how-to-cook/how-to-make-ice-cream-without-an-icecream-maker

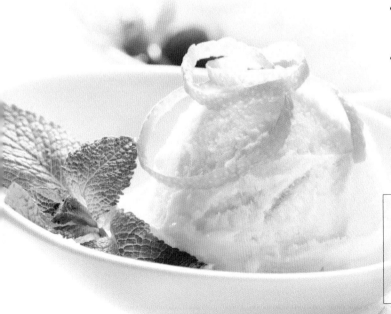

RECIPE NOTES
Adjusting and customizing the recipes

There is not a one size fits all recipe, everyone has different tastes, some have allergies and not everyone will be able to get all of the ingredients. Consider the recipes as a guideline to which you can then customize to your own taste or to what you have in the house.

• Love coconut? Try coconut milk instead of almond milk.

• Do not like strawberries? Try blueberries.

Only you know what your preferences are, so have some fun with it and play around with different ingredients and recipes.

The book is divided into chocolate, fruits and unique recipes. The fruit variants will have a slightly higher NET carb count (but still low). Do not shy away from these though, fruits contain a whole range of nutrients that are great for your overall health.

And lastly, if you would be kind enough to leave an honest review it would be most appreciated.

Please visit link below:

http://geni.us/KetoIceRev

Once again, thank you for buying' and good luck.

Elizabeth Lane

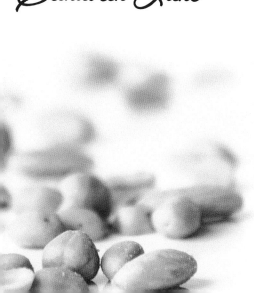

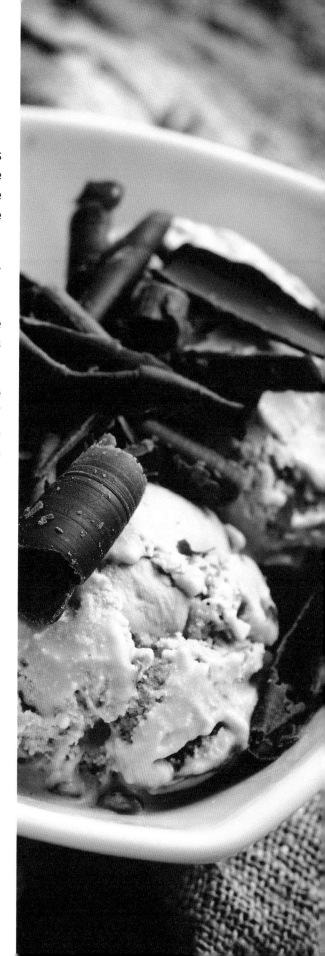

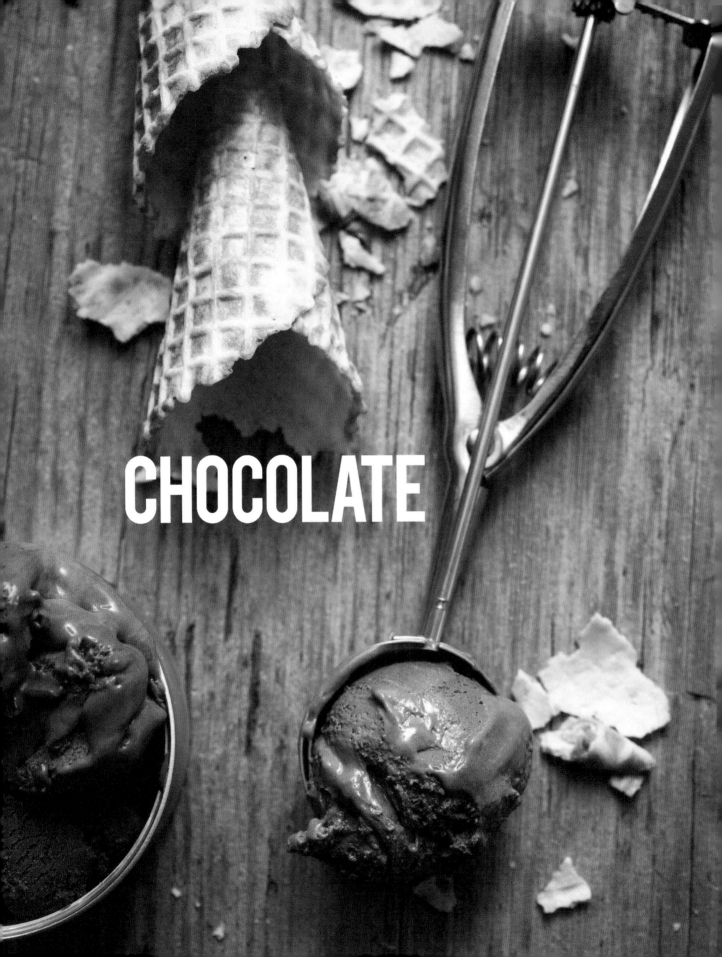

CHOCOLATE

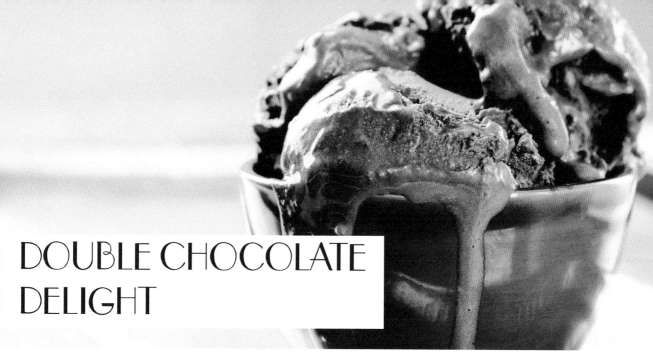

DOUBLE CHOCOLATE DELIGHT

🥄 **5 minutes**   🕐 **20 minutes**   👤 **x8**   ❄️ **3 hours**

INGREDIENTS

» 3 Ounces Dark Chocolate
» 2 Cups Heavy Cream
» 1 ½ Cups Almond Milk
» ½ Cup Erythritol
» ½ Cup Cocoa Powder
» 2 Tablespoons Glycerin
» 1 Teaspoon Scraped Vanilla Bean
» ¼ Teaspoon Xanthan Gum
» 4 Egg Yolks
» Liquid Stevia to Taste
» A Pinch of Salt

Equipment:

» Small Saucepan
» Candy Thermometer
» Whisk
» Ice Bath
» Ice Cream Maker

DIRECTIONS

1. Combine stevia, almond milk and heavy cream in your sauce pan. Whisk to combine and put on the heat.
2. In a large bowl, beat the yolks until smooth.
3. Use your candy thermometer to check the temperature of the mixture. When it reaches 170 degrees, remove from heat and pour over the yolks. Mix immediately or otherwise the yolks will scald and cook.
4. Mix evenly and then return to the saucepan and put it back on heat.
5. Prepare the ice bath.
6. When the temperature reaches 175 degrees, remove from heat and add in the chocolate. Whisk to mix until smooth and creamy.
7. Place over the ice bath and allow to sit for about 10–15 minutes then mix in the remaining ingredients.
8. Put in an ice cream maker and churn according to directions.
9. Place in the freezer for at least 2-3 hours.

Additional Tips

10. To prepare an ice bath, spread ice cubes in a shallow but wide container. Place a bowl in the middle and surround it with ice.
11. Glycerin and xanthan gum are optional but they help in achieving the right texture.

NUTRITION FACTS (PER SERVING)

Total Carbohydrates: 10g	Dietary Fiber: 3g	Net Carbs: 7g
Protein: 6g	Total Fat: 29g	Calories: 307

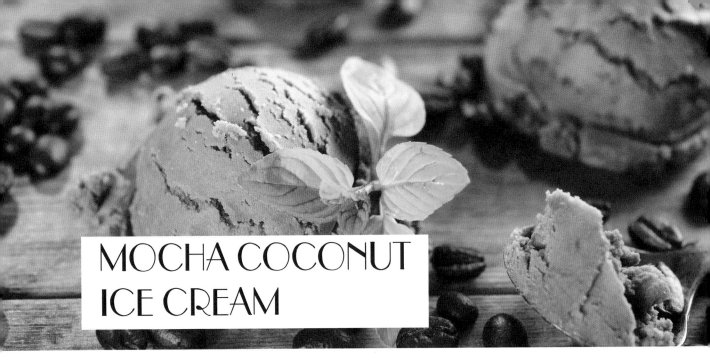

MOCHA COCONUT ICE CREAM

🥄 **5 minutes**   🕐 **-**   👤 **x8**   ❄️ **3-4 hours**

INGREDIENTS

- » 4 Cups Coconut Milk
- » 1 Cup Coconut Cream
- » 8 Tablespoons Dark Cocoa Powder
- » 4 Tablespoons Instant Coffee
- » 1 Teaspoon Xanthan Gum
- » 8 Tablespoons Erythritol
- » Liquid Stevia to Taste

Equipment:

- » Blender
- » Ice Cream Maker

DIRECTIONS

1. Combine all the ingredients apart from the gum. Blend until smooth.
2. Gradually add xanthan gum and blend until homogenous.
3. Pour into your ice cream maker and churn according to directions.
4. Scoop out and enjoy!

Additional Tips

1. You can also use brewed espresso if you want.

NUTRITION FACTS (PER SERVING)

Total Carbohydrates: 6g	Dietary Fiber: 3g	Net Carbs: 3g
Protein: 2g	Total Fat: 18g	Calories: 157

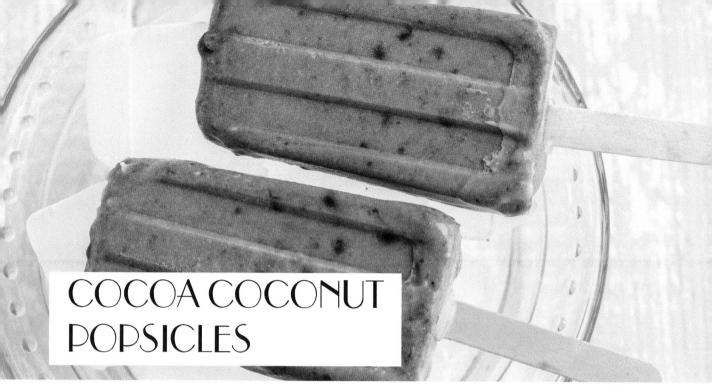

COCOA COCONUT POPSICLES

🥄 **2 minutes**   🕐 **-**   👤 **x8**   ❄️ **2 hours**

INGREDIENTS

» 13 Ounces Coconut Milk
» ⅔ Cup Cocoa Powder
» ¼ Cup Shredded Coconut
» 2 Teaspoons Vanilla Extract
» Liquid Stevia to Taste

Equipment:

» Blender
» Popsicle Molds

DIRECTIONS

1. Blend the coconut milk, cocoa powder, vanilla extract and sweetener to form a smoothie.
2. Pour into popsicle molds and freeze until set.
3. Roll in coconut flakes and enjoy!

NUTRITION FACTS (PER SERVING)

Total Carbohydrates: 5g	Dietary Fiber: 3g	Net Carbs: 2g
Protein: 2g	Total Fat: 14g	Calories: 163

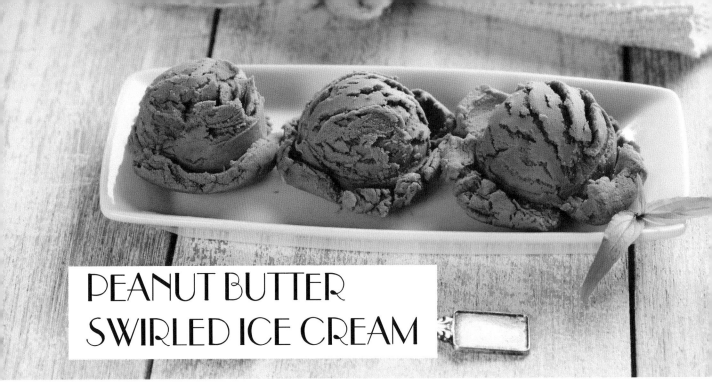

PEANUT BUTTER SWIRLED ICE CREAM

🥄 **5 minutes**   🕐 **-**   👤 **x8**   ❄️ **3-4 hours**

INGREDIENTS

- ⅔ Cup Full-Cream Milk
- 6 Tablespoons Butter
- 2 ½ Tablespoons Avocado Oil
- 2 ½ Tablespoons Cocoa Powder
- 1 ½ Teaspoons Vanilla Extract
- ¼ Teaspoon Sea Salt
- 4 Eggs
- Stevia to Taste

For the swirl:

- ⅔ Cup Peanut Butter (smooth)
- 5 Tablespoons Coconut Oil
- Stevia to Taste

Equipment:

- Blender
- Ice Cream Maker
- Whisk

DIRECTIONS

1. Crack the eggs and separate egg yolks from two of them. You need two whole eggs and two egg yolks.
2. Add all the initial ingredients to a blender and blend until smooth. Add to an ice cream maker and churn according to directions.
3. In the meanwhile, whisk together all the swirl ingredients and place in the refrigerator.
4. Just before turning off the ice cream maker, add in the swirl and let it roll for an additional minute.
5. Scoop out and enjoy!

Additional Tips

1. Top with some chopped peanuts.
2. If you don't have access to avocado oil, replace with an equal amount of MCT oil available easily at any grocery store.

NUTRITION FACTS (PER SERVING)

Total Carbohydrates: 4g	Dietary Fiber: 2g	Net Carbs: 2g
Protein: 5g	Total Fat: 32g	Calories: 311

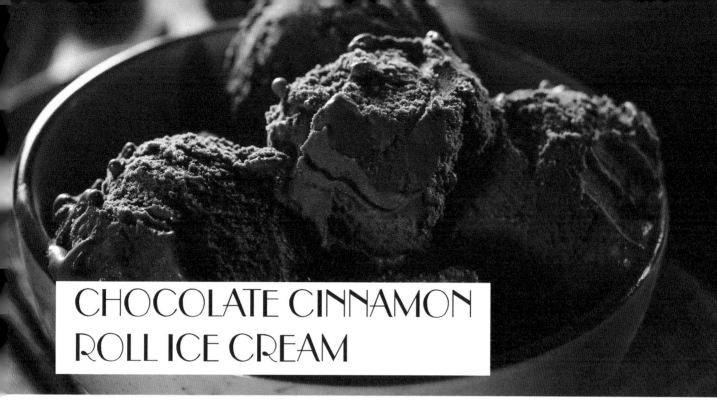

CHOCOLATE CINNAMON ROLL ICE CREAM

🥄 **2 minutes**   🕐 **-**   👤 **x8**   ❄ **3-4 hours**

INGREDIENTS

» 27 Ounces Coconut Milk
» ½ Cup Grated Dark Chocolate
» 2 Tablespoons Ground Cinnamon
» 4 Teaspoons Vanilla Extract
» 2 Teaspoons Additional Ground Cinnamon
» Erythritol to Taste

Equipment:

» Blender
» Ice Cream Maker

DIRECTIONS

1. Blend all the ingredients apart from the additional teaspoon of cinnamon.
2. Pour directly into your ice cream maker and churn until set.
3. Freeze and then scoop out and serve, sprinkling with remaining cinnamon.

Additional Tips

1. Add a splash of alcohol (preferably vodka) to prevent it from becoming too icy.

NUTRITION FACTS (PER SERVING)

Total Carbohydrates: 7g	Dietary Fiber: 2g	Net Carbs: 5g
Protein: 3g	Total Fat: 32g	Calories: 392

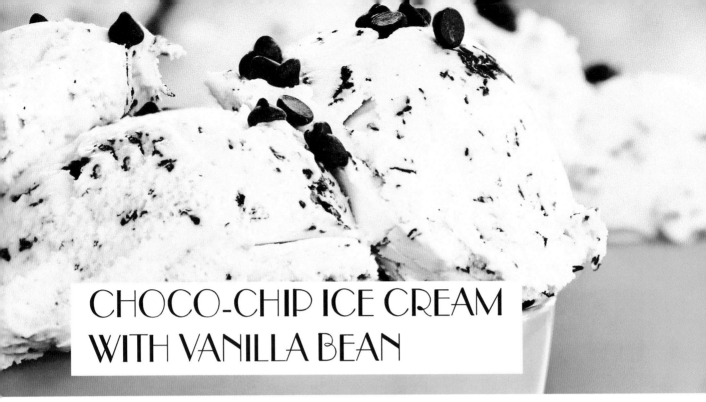

CHOCO-CHIP ICE CREAM WITH VANILLA BEAN

🥄 5 minutes   🕐 -   👤 x8   ❄ 2-3 hours

INGREDIENTS

» 2 Cups Heavy Cream
» 1 Cup Half and Half
» 1 Cup Unsweetened Chocolate Chips
» 2 Tablespoons Instant Coffee
» 1 Tablespoon Scraped Vanilla Bean
» 1 Teaspoon Glycerin
» 3 Egg Yolks
» A Pinch of Salt
» Stevia or Erythritol to Taste

Equipment:

» Blender
» Ice Cream Maker

DIRECTIONS

1. Blend all the ingredients, except the chocolate chips, until smooth.
2. Add to your ice cream maker and churn until set.
3. Just before turning it off, add in the chocolate chips and allow to run for another minute or two.
4. Scoop out and enjoy!

NUTRITION FACTS (PER SERVING)

Total Carbohydrates: 2g   Dietary Fiber: 0g   Net Carbs: 2g
Protein: 2g   Total Fat: 16g   Calories: 168

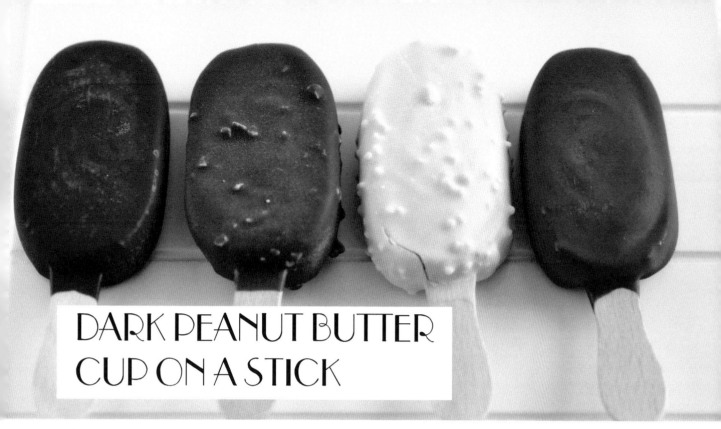

DARK PEANUT BUTTER CUP ON A STICK

🥄 **10 minutes**   🕐 **-**   👤 **x8**   ❄️ **3 hours**

INGREDIENTS

- ⅔ Cup Heavy Cream
- ⅓ Cup Full Cream Milk
- ⅓ Cup Peanut Butter (smooth)
- 1/2 Teaspoon Vanilla Extract
- Sweetener to Taste

For the Coating:

- ⅔ Cup Grated Dark Chocolate
- ⅓ Cup MCT Oil
- Sweetener to Taste

Equipment:

- Electric Beater
- Popsicle Molds
- Microwave or Double Boiler
- Parchment Paper

DIRECTIONS

1. Whip the cream until light and frothy. Your cream is done when stiff peaks form.
2. Gently fold in the rest of the ingredients.
3. Pour into molds and freeze until set.
4. In the meantime, melt together chocolate and oil over a double boiler. Mix in the sweetener and remove from heat.
5. Remove the popsicles from the freezer and dip into the chocolate mixture.
6. Set on parchment paper and return to freezer.

Additional Tips

1. Try different coatings: white chocolate, lighter chocolate or even throw in some crushed nuts.
2. Vanilla based center also works great.
3. You can also use coconut oil instead of MCT oil.

NUTRITION FACTS (PER SERVING)

Total Carbohydrates: 4g	Dietary Fiber: 0g	Net Carbs: 4g
Protein: 3g	Total Fat: 9g	Calories: 170

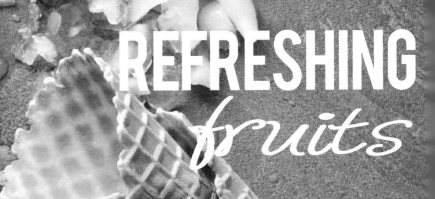

REFRESHING
fruits

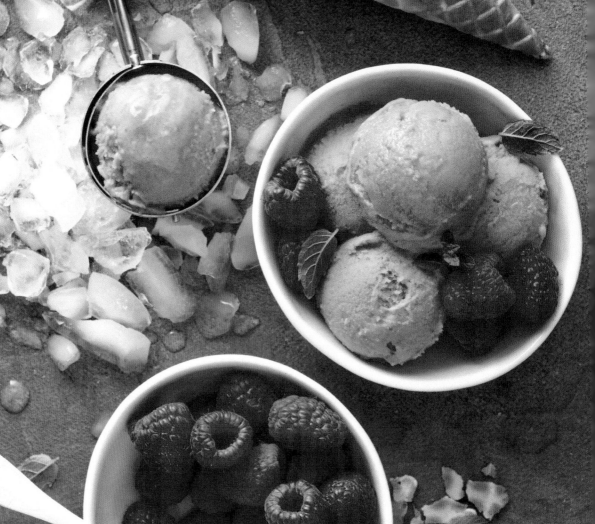

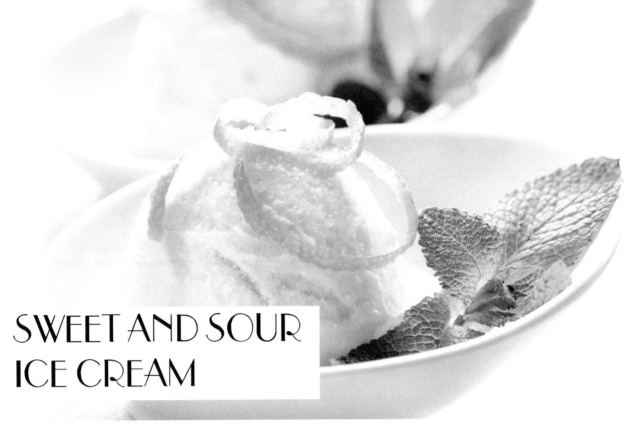

SWEET AND SOUR ICE CREAM

🥄 2 minutes   🕐 5 minutes   👤 x8   ❄️ 1 hour

INGREDIENTS

- » ⅔ Cup Fresh Lemon Juice
- » 3 Cups Full Cream Milk
- » ¾ Cup Heavy Cream
- » 2 Tablespoons Glycerin
- » 2 Tablespoons Butter
- » 1 ½ Teaspoons Vanilla Extract
- » ¼ Teaspoon Fresh Lemon Zest
- » 3 Eggs
- » A Pinch of Salt
- » Stevia to Taste
- » 2-3 Drops Yellow Food Coloring

Equipment:

- » Small Saucepan
- » Blender
- » Ice Cream Maker

DIRECTIONS

1. Blend milk, cream, lemon juice, eggs and salt until smooth.
2. Pour into a saucepan and bring to a boil.
3. When bubbles begin to appear, remove from heat and stir in the rest of the ingredients and allow to cool to room temperature.
4. Add to your ice cream maker and churn according to directions.
5. Freeze, scoop out and enjoy!

Additional Tips

1. Food coloring is optional.

NUTRITION FACTS (PER SERVING)

Total Carbohydrates: 7g	Dietary Fiber: 2g	Net Carbs: 5g
Protein: 4g	Total Fat: 13g	Calories: 154

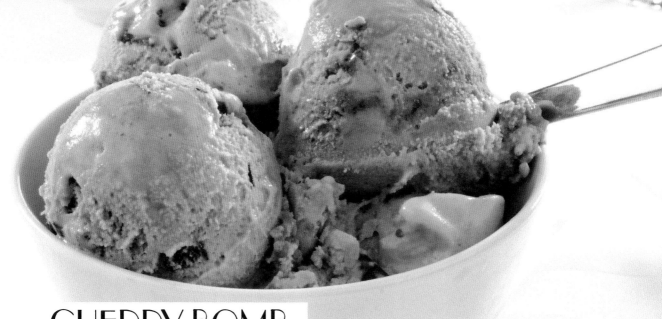

CHERRY BOMB ICE CREAM

 2 minutes   **-**   **x8**    **2-3 hours**

INGREDIENTS

- » 13.5 Ounces Coconut Milk
- » 10 Ounces Pitted Cherries
- » ½ Cup Unsweetened Chocolate Chips
- » 1 Tablespoon Glycerin
- » 1 Tablespoon Scraped Vanilla Bean
- » Erythritol to Taste

Equipment:

- » Blender
- » Ice Cream Maker

DIRECTIONS

1. Separate about 3 ounces of cherries and set aside.
2. Blend the remaining cherries, milk, sweetener and vanilla.
3. Chop the set-aside cherries and mix in by hand with the smoothie.
4. Pour into your ice cream maker and churn until set.
5. Just before turning it off, add in the chocolate chips and allow to run for one more minute.
6. Freeze, scoop and enjoy!

Additional Tips

1. Top with some sugar-free cherry syrup.

NUTRITION FACTS (PER SERVING)

Total Carbohydrates: 2g	Dietary Fiber: 0g	Net Carbs: 2g
Protein: 1g	Total Fat: 11g	Calories: 147

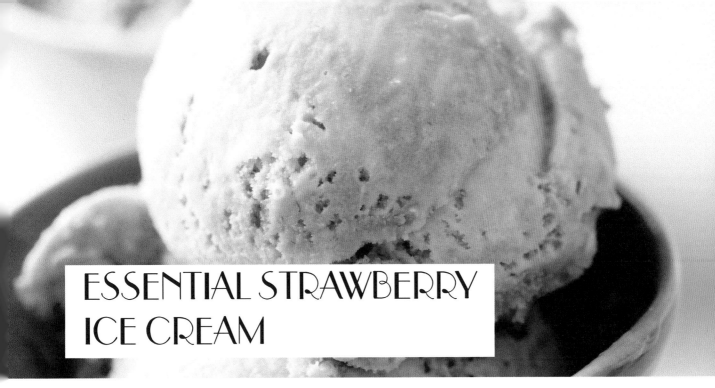

ESSENTIAL STRAWBERRY ICE CREAM

 2 minutes   **-**   **x8**    **2-3 hours**

INGREDIENTS

» 3 Cups Fresh Sliced Strawberries
» 3 Cups Full Cream Milk
» 1 Cup Heavy Cream
» ⅔ Cup Cottage Cheese
» 1 Teaspoon Vanilla Extract
» ½ Teaspoon Guar Gum
» Stevia to Taste
» A Pinch of Salt

Equipment:

» Blender
» Ice Cream Maker

DIRECTIONS

1. Blend all the ingredients until smooth.
2. Pour into your ice cream maker and churn until the desired consistency is achieved.
3. Freeze. Scoop out, top with fresh strawberries and serve.

Additional Tips

1. Just before turning the ice cream maker off, add in some chopped strawberries for added texture.
2. You can also top it with some strawberry Jell-O.

NUTRITION FACTS (PER SERVING)

Total Carbohydrates: 5g	Dietary Fiber: 1g	Net Carbs: 4g
Protein: 6g	Total Fat: 13g	Calories: 160

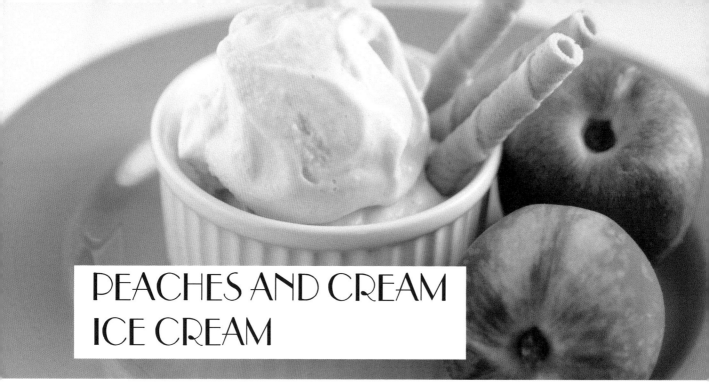

PEACHES AND CREAM ICE CREAM

🥄 **8 minutes**   🕐 **7 minutes**   👤 **x8**   ❄️ **Overnight**

INGREDIENTS

- » 3 Large Peaches
- » 2 Cups Heavy Cream
- » 1 ½ Cups Half and Half
- » ½ Cup Water
- » Erythritol to Taste
- » 2-3 Drops Orange Food Coloring

DIRECTIONS

1. Peel and dice the peaches. Puree one peach with the water and set aside.
2. Whisk together the cream, peach puree, sweetener, food coloring and half and half.
3. Pour into your ice cream maker and churn according to the directions. When the ice cream starts to firm up, add in the finely chopped peaches.
4. Freeze overnight.
5. Scoop out and enjoy!

Additional Tips

1. Add in some xanthan gum to keep the ice cream soft.

NUTRITION FACTS (PER SERVING)

Total Carbohydrates: 9g	Dietary Fiber: 4g	Net Carbs: 5g
Protein: 2g	Total Fat: 21g	Calories: 207

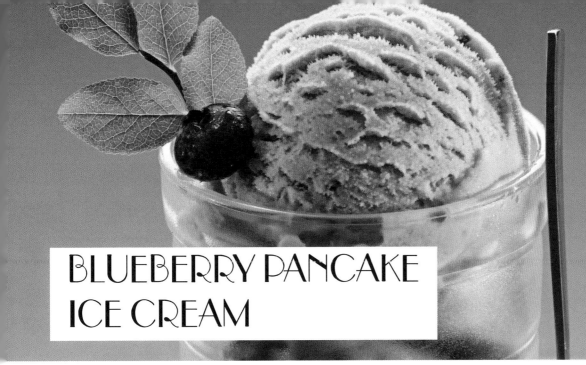

BLUEBERRY PANCAKE ICE CREAM

🥄 20 minutes   🕐 10 minutes   👤 x8   ❄ Overnight

INGREDIENTS

» 1 Cup Heavy Cream
» 1 ⅛ Cups Buttermilk
» 1 ½ Tablespoons Glycerin
» 1 Teaspoon Red Wine Vinegar
» Stevia to Taste
» A Pinch of Salt

For the puree:

» ½ Pound Blueberries
» 2 Tablespoons Fresh Lime Juice
» 1 Tablespoon Water
» ¼ Teaspoon Vanilla Extract
» ⅛ Teaspoon Almond Extract
» ⅛ Teaspoon Ground Cinnamon
» ⅛ Teaspoon Ground Nutmeg
» Stevia to Taste

Equipment:

» Immersion Blender
» Small Saucepan
» Ice Cream Maker

DIRECTIONS

1. Add the blueberries, water, lemon juice and spices from the puree ingredients list to a small saucepan.
2. Heat on low heat until softened. Mash using a wooden spoon.
3. Use an immersion blender to puree the mixture. Add the vanilla and almond extracts and stevia.
4. Cook and simmer until it becomes syrupy and thick. At any point, add a splash of water if you fear scalding. Remove from heat and cool to room temperature.
5. Add all the ingredients to your ice cream maker and churn until set.
6. Freeze, scoop out and serve.

Additional Tips

1. Balsamic vinegar reduction instead of red wine vinegar also works perfectly. To make reduced balsamic vinegar, take ¼ cup of balsamic vinegar and put it on low heat. Simmer until about half remains behind. Remove from heat and cool.

NUTRITION FACTS (PER SERVING)

Total Carbohydrates: 6g   Dietary Fiber: 1g   Net Carbs: 5g
Protein: 2g   Total Fat: 16g   Calories: 161

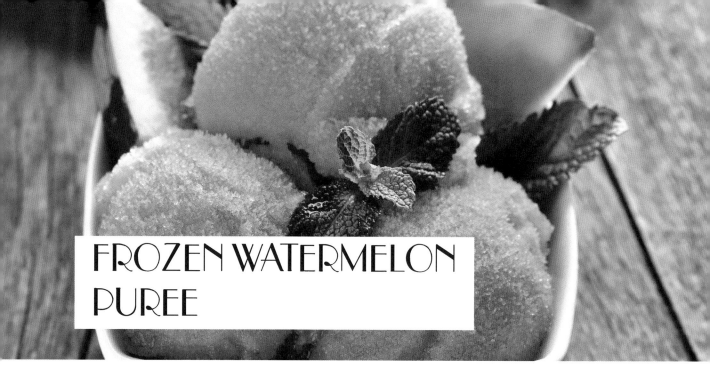

FROZEN WATERMELON PUREE

🥄 **8 minutes**   🕐 **10 minutes**   👤 **x8**   ❄️ **Overnight**

INGREDIENTS

- » 8 Cups Diced Watermelon
- » 2 Cups Coconut Milk
- » 2 Teaspoons Fresh Lemon Juice
- » Liquid Stevia to Taste

Equipment:

- » Food Processor

DIRECTIONS

1. Freeze the watermelon overnight.
2. Place the diced watermelon in your food processor and begin to mix at slow speed. It is very important to keep the speed low.
3. When it becomes icy and puree-like, add the coconut milk and the rest of the ingredients. Continue to blend while pausing in between to scrape the sides.
4. After some time, air will be incorporated in the fruit and you will have a sherbet-like consistency.
5. Scoop out and serve immediately.

Additional Tips

1. There are no intricate ingredients in this recipe. The trick is the technique. Hence you'll need a good food processor and lots of patience.

NUTRITION FACTS (PER SERVING)

Total Carbohydrates: 10g	Dietary Fiber: 2g	Net Carbs: 8g
Protein: 2g	Total Fat: 14g	Calories: 184

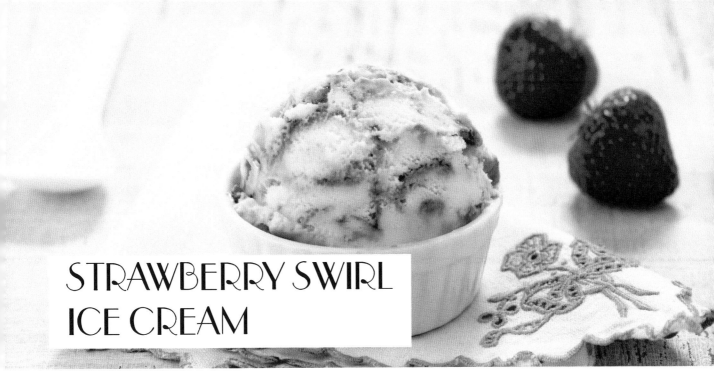

STRAWBERRY SWIRL ICE CREAM

🥄 8 minutes   🕐 40 minutes   👤 x8   ❄️ 3-4 hours

INGREDIENTS

» 1 Cup Frozen Strawberries
» 4 Ounces Cream Cheese
» 1 Cup Full Cream Milk
» 1 ¼ Cups Heavy Whipping Cream
» 2 Tablespoons Glycerin
» ½ Teaspoon Vanilla Extract
» ½ Teaspoon Xanthan Gum
» 3 Egg Yolks
» Stevia to Taste

Equipment:

» Whisk
» Small Saucepan
» Ice Bath
» Ice Cream Maker

DIRECTIONS

1. Whisk together the egg yolks until smooth and mix in the sweetener.
2. In your saucepan, mix the cream and milk. Bring to a boil.
3. Pour this over the egg yolks while continuing to whisk or otherwise they will cook. This process is called tempering.
4. Return the whole mixture to the saucepan and continue to cook on medium heat until it has a thick custard-like consistency.
5. Remove from heat and add in rest of the ingredients, except the strawberries, and set over an ice bath.
6. When cooled, pour into your ice cream maker and churn. While it is churning, mash the strawberries with some powdered erythritol or stevia. Make sure to mash into a goopy mixture. Add some water if needed.
7. Just before turning the ice cream maker off, pour in the mashed strawberries and allow to churn for about five more minutes.
8. Remove and freeze. Scoop out and enjoy.

Additional Tips

1. To learn how to prepare an ice bath, refer back to the Double Chocolate Delight recipe.
2. The consistency in step four will be perfect when the mixture evenly coats the back of a spoon.

NUTRITION FACTS (PER SERVING)

Total Carbohydrates: 4g	Dietary Fiber: 1g	Net Carbs: 3g
Protein: 4g	Total Fat: 27g	Calories: 115

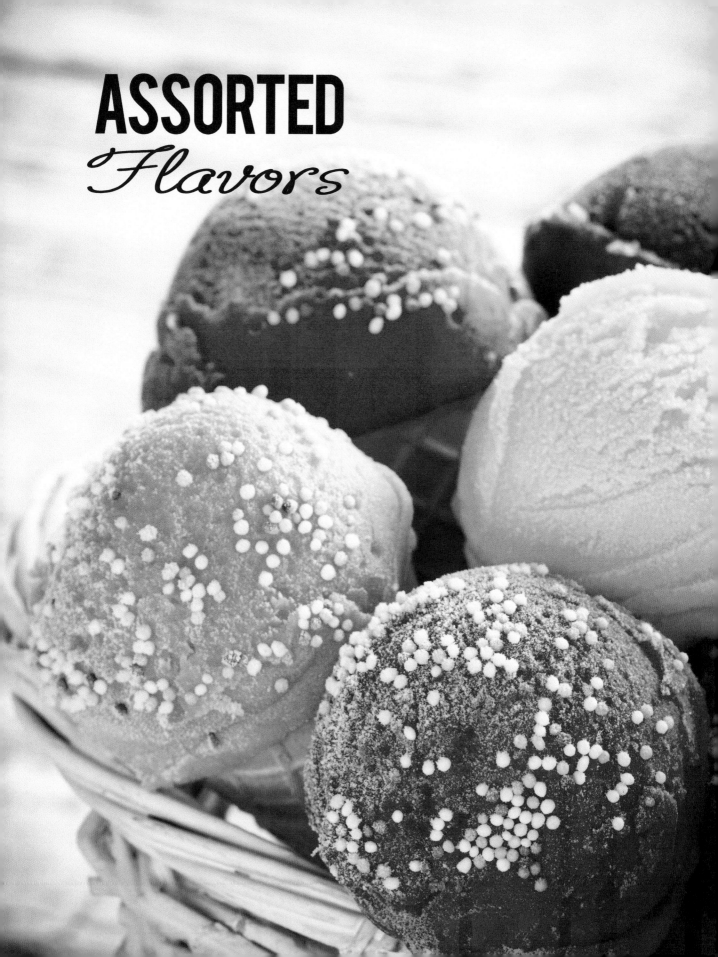

ASSORTED
Flavors

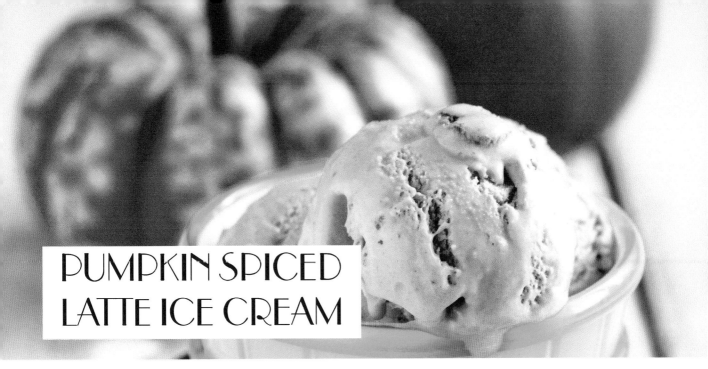

PUMPKIN SPICED LATTE ICE CREAM

🥄 2 minutes   🕐 7 minutes   👤 x8   ❄️ 3-4 hours

INGREDIENTS

» 4 Cups Full Cream Milk
» 1 Cup Pumpkin Puree
» 1 Cup Cottage Cheese
» ½ cup pumpkin seeds
» 4 Tablespoons Salted Butter
» 2 Teaspoons Maple Extract
» 1 Teaspoon Xanthan Gum
» 6 Egg Yolks
» Stevia to Taste

Equipment:

» Frying Pan
» Immersion Blender
» Ice Cream Maker

DIRECTIONS

1. Put your frying pan over medium heat and melt the butter. Add the pumpkin seeds and cook until toasted. Remove from heat and set aside.
2. Beat the egg yolks until creamy and mix in the sweetener. You can either use a liquid sweetener or a granulated one, it is up to you.
3. Pour the milk into the egg mixture and mix well.
4. Add the rest of the ingredients, except the pumpkin seeds, and mix using an immersion blender.
5. Pour into your ice cream maker and churn until set. Just before turning it off, add the pumpkin seeds and churn for another 3–5 minutes.
6. Freeze, scoop out and enjoy!

Additional Tips

1. Pumpkin seeds might not be to everyone's tastes, try crushed nuts or choc-chips.

NUTRITION FACTS (PER SERVING)

Total Carbohydrates: 7g	Dietary Fiber: 2g	Net Carbs: 5g
Protein: 6g	Total Fat: 27g	Calories: 271

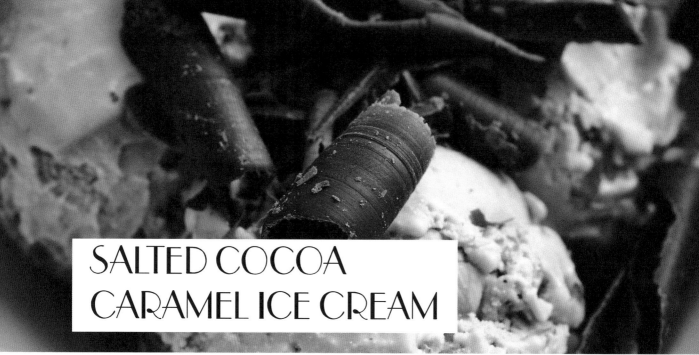

SALTED COCOA CARAMEL ICE CREAM

 10 minutes    **2 minutes**   **x8**    **2-3 hours**

INGREDIENTS

» 3 Ounces Unsweetened Dark Chocolate Chips
» 1 ½ Cups Heavy Whipping Cream
» 1 Cup Full Cream Milk
» 6 Tablespoons Butter
» 2 Tablespoons Coconut Sugar
» 2 Tablespoons Glycerin
» ¾ Teaspoon Sea Salt
» ½ Teaspoon Vanilla Extract
» ¼ Teaspoon Xanthan Gum
» 4 Egg Yolks
» Stevia to Taste

Equipment:
» Small Saucepan
» Whisk
» Candy Thermometer
» Ice Cream Maker
» Ice Bath

DIRECTIONS

1. In your saucepan, combine butter, coconut sugar and stevia. Put on low heat and bring the mixture to a boil. Continue to stir. Remove from heat and stir in the salt and vanilla. Return to heat.
2. Add in cream while stirring continuously. When the cream mixture reaches 170 degrees, whisk in milk.
3. In a small bowl, beat the egg yolks until smooth. You'll be tempering the egg yolks like we did earlier. Pour the milk mixture over egg yolks while whisking continuously to prevent scalding.
4. Return this mixture to the saucepan and put back on heat. Maintain temperature at 180 degrees. Cook until it thickens enough to coat the spoon evenly.
5. Remove from heat and set over an ice bath. Stir in glycerin and xanthan gum.
6. When cooled to room temperature, pour into your ice cream maker and churn until set.

Additional Tips

1. Only a coarse salt like kosher salt or sea salt will work. Regular table salt won't enhance the flavor like we want it to.

NUTRITION FACTS (PER SERVING)

Total Carbohydrates: 8g   Dietary Fiber: 1g   Net Carbs: 7g

Protein: 3g   Total Fat: 29g   Calories: 326

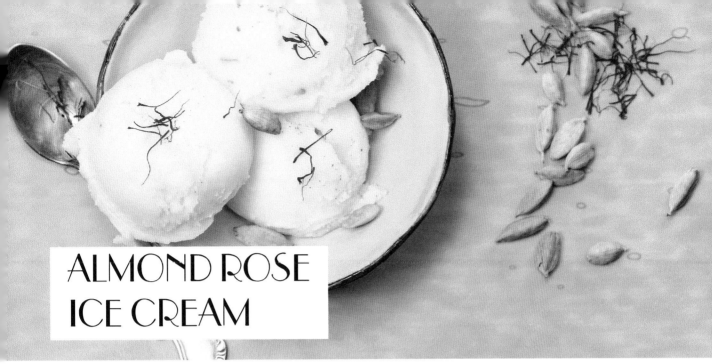

ALMOND ROSE ICE CREAM

🥄 **10 minutes**　🕐 **-**　👤 **x8**　❄️ **6-7 hours**

INGREDIENTS

- » 2 Cups Heavy Whipping Cream
- » 1 Cup Almond Milk
- » ½ Cup Unsweetened Rose Petal Paste
- » ½ Cup Raw Almonds
- » 4 Tablespoons Rose Water
- » Erythritol to Taste

Equipment:
- » Food Processor
- » Electric Beater

DIRECTIONS

1. Soak the almonds in water overnight. Peel them and set aside in the morning.
2. Drain the water and pat dry with a paper towel.
3. Powder in food processor as finely as possible. You might need to pause and scrape the sides a few times.
4. Beat the cream until stiff peaks form. Add in the milk and beat again.
5. Fold in the rest of the ingredients.
6. Scoop out into a metallic container and place in the freezer.
7. After two hours, the ice cream should be solidified. Stir it thoroughly and return to the freezer. After a further two hours, stir the ice cream again and return to freezer. Do this three times.
8. Scoop out and serve.

Additional Tips
1. You can easily find rose petal paste at any Indian specialty store.
2. For simplicity, you can also just add the mixture to an ice cream maker and churn until done but I wanted to show an alternate method for people who might not have an ice cream maker.
3. Since there are no softening agents such as xanthan gum in the recipe, the ice cream will freeze solid if left for longer periods. Hence it being best consumed fresh. However if you have some left over, soften it a little by transferring to the fridge for a little while before serving.

NUTRITION FACTS (PER SERVING)

Total Carbohydrates: 5g	Dietary Fiber: 1g	Net Carbs: 4g
Protein: 1g	Total Fat: 14g	Calories: 175

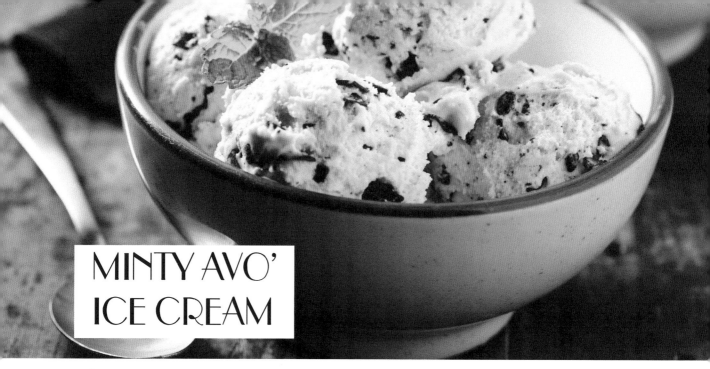

MINTY AVO' ICE CREAM

🥄 **20 minutes**   🕐 **-**   👤 **x8**   ❄️ **Overnight**

INGREDIENTS

- » 4 Bananas
- » 2 Avocados
- » ⅔ Cup Cocoa Nibs
- » ½ Teaspoon Xanthan Gum
- » ¼ Teaspoon Peppermint Extract
- » Stevia to Taste

Equipment:

- » Food Processor

DIRECTIONS

1. Freeze the bananas overnight. Slice them into rounds.
2. Peel and dice the avocados.
3. Place both the avocados and the bananas in a food processor.
4. Blend on low. Pause frequently to scrape the sides. Due to the frozen bananas, the mixture will start to get a mousse-like consistency. Keep blending until the mixture becomes light and frothy.
5. Stir in the rest of the ingredients then transfer to the freezer and freeze for a couple of hours.
6. Scoop out and serve.

Additional Tips

1. Add some cocoa powder to instantly make this into chocolate ice cream.
2. You can easily store it in the freezer for prolonged periods but due to the bananas, it might brown a little.

NUTRITION FACTS (PER SERVING)

Total Carbohydrates: 11g	Dietary Fiber: 6g	Net Carbs: 5g
Protein: Less than 1g	Total Fat: 10g	Calories: 183

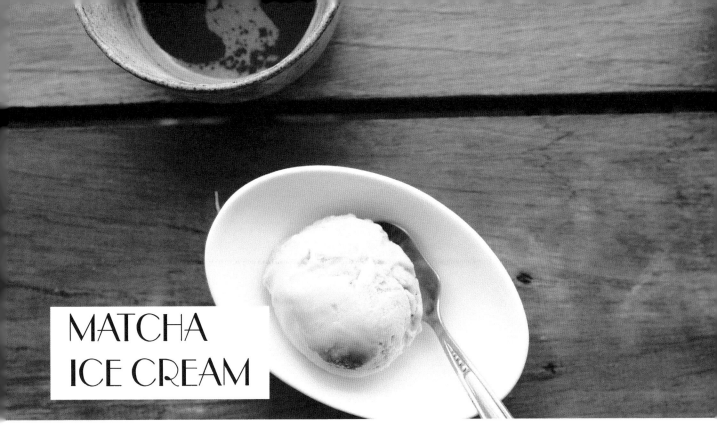

MATCHA ICE CREAM

🥄 **2 minutes**　　🕐 **5 minutes**　　👤 **x8**　　❄️ **2-3 hours**

INGREDIENTS

» 27 Ounces Coconut Milk
» 3 Tablespoons Coconut Oil
» 2 Tablespoons Matcha Green Tea Powder
» ¼ Teaspoon Guar Gum
» Stevia to Taste

Equipment:
» Small Saucepan
» Ice Bath
» Ice Cream Maker

DIRECTIONS

1. Pour coconut milk into your saucepan and set over low heat.
2. Add in the matcha green tea powder and begin to stir. Do not allow to boil.
3. When completely dissolved, (the milk will turn green) pour into a bowl and set over the ice bath.
4. Stir in rest of the ingredients.
5. When cooled to room temperature, pour into your ice cream maker and churn until set.
6. Freeze, scoop and enjoy.

Additional Tips

1. Do not make the mistake of using regular green tea. You can find matcha green tea at Whole Foods, Trader Joe's and even on Amazon.

NUTRITION FACTS (PER SERVING)

Total Carbohydrates: 5g	Dietary Fiber: 2g	Net Carbs: 3g
Protein: 2g	Total Fat: 28g	Calories: 264

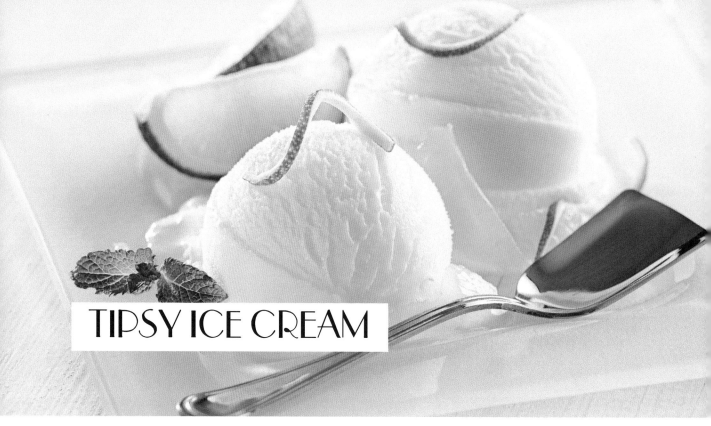

TIPSY ICE CREAM

🥄 **5 minutes**   🕐 **-**   👤 **x8**   ❄️ **3-4 hours**

INGREDIENTS

- » 2 Cups Full Cream Milk
- » 2 Cups Half and Half
- » 1 ⅓ Cups Lime Juice
- » 4-6 Tablespoons Silver Tequila
- » 2 Tablespoons Lime Zest
- » Stevia to Taste

Equipment:
- » Blender
- » Ice Cream Maker

DIRECTIONS

1. Add all the ingredients to a high-speed blender and blend until smooth and creamy.
2. Pour into your ice cream maker and churn until desired consistency is achieved.
3. Freeze, scoop and enjoy!

Additional Tips
1. The milk will curdle due to the sour lime juice. Don't worry, it is totally normal and won't affect the outcome in any negative way.

NUTRITION FACTS (PER SERVING)

Total Carbohydrates: 8g	Dietary Fiber: 4g	Net Carbs: 4g
Protein: 3g	Total Fat: 23g	Calories: 145

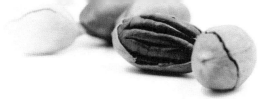

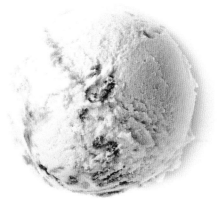
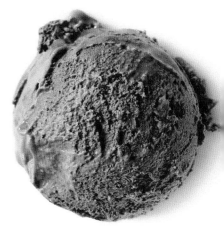
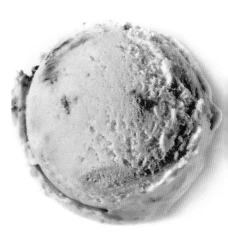
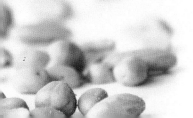

Printed in Great
Britain
by Amazon

31876677R00017